M.E. and Me

A Doctor's Struggle with Chronic

Fatigue Syndrome

Dr KN Hng

ISBN-13: 978-1974267507

ISBN-10: 1974267504

Facebook group – Dr Hng's ME/CFS Friends:
https://www.facebook.com/groups/113427572678279/

Email: RColourMusic@hotmail.com

eStore: https://www.createspace.com/7431027

Also on Amazon.

Music books: https://www.facebook.com/RColourMusic/

Dedication

This book is dedicated to all ME/CFS sufferers, a misunderstood, neglected and forgotten group of patients, many of whom have died in the absence of the help we need, and/or suffered further damage from incorrect, harmful treatments.

This YouTube video makes a beautiful dedication:
https://www.youtube.com/watch?v=IOflARSgNnE& feature=youtu.be

Preface

I have a story to tell. There are many things in here which I am not at all comfortable sharing, yet I want to tell the whole story. Therefore I have decided to share them. I hope doing so will help educate, inform, and raise awareness. From my own experience, both as a doctor and then as a patient, this condition is poorly understood. After all, isn't *everyone* tired all the time?

CONTENTS

Not Good Enough

I was a doctor. A busy, National Health Service, very senior Junior Doctor. Then I became ill with ME / Chronic Fatigue Syndrome.

I was struggling desperately for months, even years. Failing to perform at work, being told I was slow in clinic, I wasn't showing leadership, I didn't carry myself like a Consultant, etc. I was just so exhausted all the time, I barely managed to do the minimum. I drank more, and more, and MORE coffee, squeezing every last ounce of energy out of my poor tired body.

For being "not good enough", I got more things thrown at me. More work-based assessments, more appraisals, more meetings, more portfolio activity, in addition to the usual courses, fifteen-hundred-word assignments, and teaching presentations to prepare, which only added to my load.

So I tried harder. Soooo hard. Staying up late every night working on all that was asked, fighting sleep. Investing hours into teaching activities, and speeding through clinics. Working relentlessly through the grueling 12.5 hour Long Day and Night shifts, pushing through the exhaustion.

I clocked up as many as nine patients in a clinic, dosed up on coffee and running on sheer willpower. I managed Consultant clinics on my own (the Consultant had suddenly taken ill, and sadly never returned).

Yet no matter what I did, it was never enough. My training time was extended as I had not proven myself able to take on the heavy workload and responsibilities of a Consultant.

A Desperate Struggle

One night shift, I just couldn't drag myself off the chair in the office. My whole body had turned to lead, an enormous weight, and my head was glued to the desk. All I could do was answer bleeps/pages and questions from the neglected Junior House Officer. With great difficulty, forcing my head and arms to move and work the telephone.

That was flagged up. It was serious. And I took desperate measures. Like paying for a hotel when on Nights just to try to sleep and perform better, and my child frequently missing her bath to reduce the strain. My boss referred me for hypnotherapy.

In desperation, I took myself to see the Occupational Health doctor. For the first time I was able to express how I struggled, yet failed. A fact that so far had to be hidden, in my efforts to prove myself capable. I dissolved into tears.

~~~~~~~

Following that visit, I was commenced on an anti-depressant. And then had to deal with terrible side effects. Now on top of everything else, I suffered severe constipation and juggled insane amounts of time in the toilet, feeling permanently bloated, gaining weight and draining my time and energy even further. (sobs!)

My shifts were cut back slightly, but I didn't improve. It just slowed my decline. After a Long Day (12.5 hrs), I would be absolutely shattered all the next day, which I accepted as normal. But on the second and third days, I still felt exactly the same, as if I had been on-call the day before.

By this point, I was in constant mild pain. All my muscles were stiff and every movement ached, as if I had run a marathon the previous day. These symptoms were permanent but became much worse after on-call shifts. And still I didn't know I was ill.

On the fourth and fifth days I would feel only a tiny bit better. I still fought exhaustion, ached with every movement, and struggled to excel. When the next on-call shift came around, I still hadn't recovered. At the end of one shift I must have looked ghastly, for a colleague exclaimed when he saw me, "Now that's a broken woman!"

~~~~~~~

Getting up in the morning required superhuman effort. I began to set my alarm to an earlier time to give myself longer to get ready. I wasn't safe driving. Not only did I fall asleep driving home from work, I struggled to keep awake driving in! The 1.5 hour commute made things worse. A "short day" would be 12 hours long. I was constantly worried that I would die in a car crash and leave my children orphaned.

Once home, I would collapse onto the couch for half an hour or more. This upset my children, who had been looking forward to seeing me, so my husband and I determined that I should park up somewhere and rest in the car before returning to the house. I deteriorated further, and then I was sleeping in the car park at the hospital before driving home, for I could not face the journey.

After Long Days, as badly as I needed it, I was too exhausted to manage a shower. A change of clothes had to do.

It's Not Depression!

On the 29th June 2016, six months after that fateful night shift, I couldn't carry on any longer. I will never forget that day. I went to my GP, burst into tears again, and cried, "I don't feel safe!" I knew if I carried on I'd kill somebody.

Sobbing uncontrollably again earned me yet another anti-depressant. This time it made me stop eating, and I became very weak as a result. When I realised what had happened, I threw the rest out. I couldn't afford to be made even more ill, and I was still reeling from the side effects of the last one!

With the first anti-depressant, I had persevered for over two months, knowing it takes time to have an effect. I didn't feel depressed, but I was so desperate for an explanation, for someone to know what to do, I was willing to try anything. And I had a totally dreadful experience, whilst also fighting my losing battle at work. Even after discontinuing the tablets, it was many months before I was less bloated, and a total of six months before I felt properly back to normal.

I never felt depressed, even with all that I was going through. I have always had a positive outlook on life, with a tendency to err on the side of optimism. At work, I never doubted I could make it, despite everything. Even at home, lying on the sofa with my eyes shut because I was so ill, I was happy. I delighted in the precious sound of my children playing, and felt so glad to be resting at last!

I was finally diagnosed at the specialist ME clinic. They confirmed I wasn't depressed. I was thoroughly screened for depression, anxiety and sleep apnoea, scoring near zero for all of them. The specialist said, "Just because you cry doesn't mean you're depressed."

Run Into the Ground

Life was UTTER HELL before I went off sick. I wanted so desperately to stay home and sleep, yet I had no "reason" to be off work, no "illness", and there wasn't anything obviously wrong with me. Just being exhausted was not an acceptable reason. Instead, it was the accepted norm!

As a doctor, you work the rotas, relentless and unsustainable as they are. AND sit exams, maintain your portfolio, attend courses, prepare teaching resources, and undertake extra projects such as audit, quality improvement, or write up research for publication, all in your own time, just to prove yourself competent and employable at the end of your training. Meanwhile the rotas become more and more punishing, as staffing levels drop unmanageably due to changes in government policy.

At the end of 2013, I returned to work following a prolonged absence on maternity and sick leave. I failed miserably. My boss asked me, "What's wrong with you?" but I didn't have an answer for him. I never let him know how I struggled to stay awake in clinic, sometimes even whilst speaking to a patient. I believed I was simply "unfit" after my prolonged absence. I was so ashamed of it, I was unable to share the secret.

That was the start of the escalating doses of coffee.

Over the next two years, my performance and competency improved significantly, with sheer determination and grit. I excelled at teaching, I needed little supervision, and my specialist knowledge increased steadily. I received brilliant patient feedback and got many competencies signed off.

But I did not shine. It took all I had to execute the

work. I did not have the energy to lead, nor the strength to rise to Consultant level performance. I was so exhausted, I didn't even have the energy to smile at people.

In the end, I ran myself into the ground. I worked to the point of collapse, vainly trying to be the superwoman that doctors who dare to have children are required to be. The situation was extreme beyond belief. I was forced to neglect my own physical needs, I self-medicated with sedatives in order to sleep at unnatural hours when on Nights, and I barely saw my children.

The sad fact is that being a doctor in the National Health Service is so demanding that I couldn't even recognise I was ill. Exhaustion just seemed normal, for everyone else was tired too. Instead of seeking help, I felt ashamed, and just pushed myself harder. "Helpful" appraisals and recommendations aimed at improving my performance just added to my load, my supervisors also failing to notice that I was ill.

For all of us in the NHS, seeing a colleague look exhausted is a normal daily occurrence. We all feel that way ourselves on a regular basis, and we can't offer much support, as we are all stretched to the limit. We don't listen to our bodies – we don't have the option to. If we did, the service would collapse and God forbid, the government would have to increase spending on staffing levels!

Living with ME/CFS

I am largely housebound. My energy levels are minimal, and dip even further if I do too much. I only shower every two or three days. This spares some energy for other activities. I brush my teeth only once each day, for by the time I have got my children dressed, done some tidying or done some work at the computer in the morning, I am spent. My husband has bought me an electric toothbrush – brushing my teeth is hard work. I have to nap and spend two hours or more in bed every day. Four hours is not uncommon.

My hair only gets washed when it is actually disgusting, and sometimes my husband washes it for me. I am not able to bathe my children – I don't have the energy. A year ago when I first came off work, I used to make an effort to do that. Then during my first therapy session at the specialist clinic,

I admitted that I had to choose between bathing my children and having my own shower. The realisation brought painful tears, again. Life was just such a losing battle!

I move slowly. Sometimes VERY slowly. I am stiff and ache all over. Apparently this is because my muscles don't have the ATP molecules required to clear away the lactic acid build-up from even the minimal activity that I do. If I get ill, all my joints seize up as well, so that even shifting my weight becomes laboured torture, all of me as stiff as a piece of wood. When the stiffness and heaviness overwhelms, I crawl on the floor, step after painful step.

The fatigue is absolutely debilitating. It is more than just feeling lacklustre. It is an all-consuming feeling of the body, head and limbs having turned into lead, and carrying the weight of stone. When gripped by it, it is a struggle even to move a finger, or to speak.

So you can't call or text a friend. You suffer alone.

At other times I simply feel exhausted, having done only an hour or less of very light activity. All my muscles are sore and I am overcome by an overwhelming need to lie down and shut my eyes. Many times I have fallen asleep, leaving the children to their own devices.

~~~~~~~

After my daily naps I wake paralysed, stuck in the netherworld between wakefulness and sleep, completely unable to move. My eyes stay shut and my body stays still. I am mentally submerged in ten feet of water – my own Netherland.

Beneath ten feet down, the water is completely murky and impenetrable. I am asleep. At just under ten feet, there appears a vague awareness of the outside world. Here I drift, near the bottom, sometimes sinking back again into oblivion.

Very slowly, I drift up out of the depths. I become more and more aware of sounds and where I am as I rise, but until I reach shallow areas, complex thoughts do not penetrate and I remain completely paralysed, my body feeling like a dead weight.

Meanwhile, my heart starts pounding uncomfortably. It is as if it's the engine that powers the process of waking up, for this happens every time. It carries on for a long period, often until after I am out of bed. When thoughts eventually penetrate, I am mostly wishing the pounding palpitations will stop.

When I reach the surface, I can finally open my eyes, and properly process sensory input from the outside world. I can't tell you how long I am stuck in the netherworld – I am not able to look at the clock until I am out of it.

Once my mind is out of Netherland, I must wait for the stone weight to lift from my body. I might be able to turn in bed, but it is another hour before I can get out of bed, and for a further hour or two, I can do no more than just sit in a chair, struggling to move even an arm. If I try to get up too soon, I discover how heavy my body is still, and fall back into bed again.

~~~~~~~~

The specialist clinic calls this the Slow Start. Other symptoms include sudden near-fainting spells on standing, ventricular ectopics (a type of palpitations that has been recorded on tape), frequent sore throats with painful lymph glands, and multiple other infections. I also get fasciculations – where a small piece of muscle randomly decides to take on a life of its own and do a little jig. This lasts minutes or happens repeatedly, which is extremely distracting.

When I am tired, I develop word-finding difficulties. Words get replaced with variably (or not!) related ones. Yesterday "glass" became "paper".

It's not that I don't know the right words. I do, and I find them within seconds when I stop and concentrate, but during speech they do not come quickly enough and others take their place. This normally automatic process becomes hard work, as if my brain functions cease when energy is in short supply. Yesterday I settled for "window". "Glass" would have come if I had tried harder, but "window" did the job.

Some patients describe severe intolerance to light and sound. I don't like bright windows when I'm tired, and I find it impossible to concentrate on my work if anybody is talking, watching videos or listening to music in the room. The cognitive load is simply too great then. Sound demands too much of the available brainpower, literally wearing me out!

Reading is a real struggle. I can read leaflets, and just about manage single articles if they are not too long, but I can't read books at all, not even middle grade children's books. At the beginning, I tried to read a guide book by ME/CFS specialist Dr Sarah Myhill, but never got past the first two chapters, even in tiny installments. Reading requires immense concentration. When I persisted through one chapter of a novel, I became very ill for days.

When my preschooler was referred to the Clumsy Children's Clinic for an unusual number of falls and bruises, I wanted to see if her heel-toe walk had improved from her first attempt at the doctor's surgery. I got up to show her what to do – and was shocked to discover I was even more unsteady than she was, completely unable to execute the walk! With a sinking feeling, I realised that my wide based gait isn't just because of general weakness and stiffness, but is due to the neurological consequences of the disease.

~~~~~~~

I react unpredictably to ordinary stresses. Emotional or psychological strain of any sort literally turns me into jelly. Shouting at the children, a phone call to the insurance company, having to rush for something, and even recounting my awful struggles makes my whole body feel weak and wobbly, making bed rest a necessary recourse.

This reaction is bewildering. For "activity" relates only to the physical, in most people's minds. However, in ME/CFS, all activity must be taken into account – physical, mental, social, emotional and psychological. Energy usage must be allowed for accordingly, or it runs out. Sufferers are taught to avoid any people or situations which are a drain on their energy.

The clinic gave one explanation which did make some sense. All the stress hormones, such as cortisol and adrenaline, and the resulting increase in metabolic rate, consume a lot of energy. This isn't noticeable when a person is healthy and wakes up with 100 energy chips every day, but has a profound effect when one wakes up with only five!

~~~~~~~

Energy chips – that's how I think of the problem. A normal person wakes up with 100 chips in the morning if they have had a very good night. Most days they will wake up with about 95 chips, or 90 if they've had a very busy week. Even if they were ill or were out drinking until 3 o'clock in the morning, they will not dip below 70 chips.

I wake up with just 5 or 6 chips. With this, I have to get through my day. If I have a shower, I use up one chip. Washing my hair doubles that. If I experience any emotional or psychological stress, another chip or two is spent. Filling in a 50-page social benefit form consumes four chips!

I never know for sure how I'm going to be from one day to the next. Making plans is impossible. If I have been doing too much, I wake up with just 2 or 3 chips. On days like that, I have to spend many hours in bed. When I have a crash, I have to get by on just ONE miserable chip!

How Bad Can It Get?

After going off sick, I needed to have my thyroid function, blood count, vitamin and iron levels, inflammatory markers and liver and kidney functions checked, along with a test for Epstein Barr Virus. So ignoring the desire for sleep, I drove to the phlebotomist, sitting with my eyes shut in the waiting room. I didn't know then what I know now. I felt abnormally tired, but accepted it as part of my likely diagnosis – ME/CFS, not knowing how damaging it was to push through when I needed rest. I thought nothing of driving exhausted, as I had been driving to and from work until just two days before.

That day, I became so ill I couldn't get out of bed. To get to the toilet, I had to lean against the walls, doors and chair, and my knees wobbled from being so weak. Standing up made my head woozy.

It was frightening. I worried it might be Guillain Barre Syndrome (recent multiple severe and systemically debilitating sore throats), or Myasthenia Gravis (fatiguability).

The doctor examined me, testing my muscle power. The effort of flexing my muscles for him left me shaking, even lying in bed, I was so weak. I was left bedridden for two days.

~~~~~~~

There have been multiple crashes. Life seemed to be a cycle of becoming severely debilitated, and then taking 6 weeks to get just a little strength back. I would then attempt to build myself back up by going for walks round my little cul de sac, only to quickly crash again. Each crash was a crushing disappointment, made harder by the fact that I could not know what to expect. I would think I'd be better after two or three days, but find that I was still just as ill after two weeks.

Over time, I learnt how severely I must restrict my activities in order to maintain a stable baseline. I also learnt how much energy non-physical things consume. Cold weather, having visitors, and the children being off school all take their toll. Emotional and psychological stresses had to be brought under control.

I learnt to better understand and interpret how I feel. Where early on I would have thought, "I'm feeling lazy today", and proceeded to spend the day doing something sedentary, I now know it means I have done too much, and need complete rest until I feel better, or I will suffer a full crash. That means avoiding even mental exertion, and it does not guarantee I will not crash.

It is a very different mindset for someone who has never before been allowed to "feel lazy".

~~~~~~~

The last time I crashed, I went five days without a shower. I got out of bed only to eat and to use the bathroom. Getting to the kitchen was a mammoth task. Every step and stumble was a fight, everything hurt, and I felt a hundred years old. Day and night I was in bed, alone. It so happened that everyone had gone to my in-laws' for the week. For that I was glad, as I did not want my children to see me in such a frightening state.

After so many cycles of crashing and recovering painfully slowly, it was soul-destroying for it to happen yet again, when I had been so careful with my activity levels. I felt I had no control. I was terrified that I would never get better, that I would wither away and die. I was afraid that I would never again be the clever doctor who helps people. I was heartbroken about all the things I couldn't do with my children, and I mourned all the losses if I should die.

After five days, I finally managed to have a shower and wash my hair. I had to do it sitting on the floor, and shampoo my hair twice because it was in such a state. Afterwards, I was so exhausted I had to lie in bed for two hours, desperately trying not to fall asleep, before I gained the strength to brush my hair. Then I couldn't fight it any longer. Sleep took me – I couldn't brush my teeth.

Thankfully by the end of the week, I had improved a little. I could move like an eighty-year-old instead of a hundred – very slowly, but manageable if I held on to the banister, walls and furniture. Hallelujah! I was relieved that my children didn't have to be frightened seeing me.

My Take on Sleep

A doctor once said to me that "unrefreshing sleep" is the hallmark of ME/CFS. Having lived through this, I believe it's not that sleep is unrefreshing, but rather that sufferers need so much sleep they just don't get enough to feel refreshed.

In the beginning, I suffered what must have sounded like "unrefreshing sleep" to a doctor. I woke up in the morning feeling shattered, muscles screaming and brain protesting, just as I had felt when I went to bed at night. It was as if the night's sleep hadn't happened, even though it had. Doctors dealing with ME/CFS patients must hear repeatedly, "I feel like I haven't slept at all."

After several months, I started to feel as if I had slept. I still became tired again very quickly, but for a short period after sleeping, I did feel better. And my theory on it is this:

ME/CFS sufferers have a very large sleep deficit and need to catch up on it before sleep starts to feel refreshing.

Put it this way: If you need 200 hours of sleep, eight or ten hours isn't going to make you feel any better. The only answer is to sleep, and sleep some more, until you have caught up.

After a night's sleep, you will have only just clocked up your normal daily requirement under ordinary circumstances, which may be six or seven hours, or as many as nine. That means you may have banked one hour towards your enormous deficit of 200 hours. That is why you need naps in the day and very long nights.

I present this as an alternative perspective on the "unrefreshing sleep". I think it is important because thinking of it this way encourages the right management – sleep your way towards recovery, not just accept it as an inevitable feature of the illness. Perhaps rather than "unrefreshing sleep", it should be called "relatively insufficient sleep"!

I would not be surprised if chronic severe sleep deprivation is eventually found to be a major risk factor for developing ME/CFS, such as that experienced by healthcare workers and shift workers. In my opinion, if you feel like sleeping, you should sleep, whatever the time of day, because you cannot improve until you have rectified your sleep deficit.

Many ME/CFS sufferers are afflicted by insomnia or poor quality sleep as well, and may need specific help for that. However, what is thought to be poor quality sleep may actually only be insufficient sleep.

When Mummy Is Ill

My little girl has been stuck in the house all day with me. She has already had to watch a DVD while I had a nap. She thinks that is a treat, but now she's dying to go out and play on her balance bicycle.

I'm in a Slow Start. I just want to lie on the sofa. Everything is so heavy, such an effort to move. The thought of balancing on a stool, which my husband has bought for this purpose, makes me want to lie down even more!

But I love my child. So I grab some pillows and cushions, and sit down on the curb, leaning against a neighbour's garden wall.

I look odd. Eyebrows rise. When neighbours come out of their homes, I do not go over to chat. I do not have the strength, so I stay firmly on my bottom.

But my daughter is happy. She zooms up and down the street, her little legs going like the clappers. She runs up a neighbour's steep drive, and flies back down on her bicycle, right across the road and into the opposite pavement. She is delighted to show me how fast she can go, and I am thrilled to get to see it.

~~~~~~~

Another day and I don't even have the strength to sit leaning against the wall. So I lay a mat down on my drive, settle with my cushions, and lie down with a cloth over my face. I try to look up every so often to check that my little girl is ok. Fortunately she spends a lot of time cycling in little circles around me. The slope on our drive is fun for her too. I pretend the neighbours think I'm sunbathing, even though nobody does it on their front drive.

~ ~ ~ ~ ~ ~ ~

Sometimes when I am on my own with her, my little girl says to me, "Mummy, you go and rest now. I want a video."

When I offered to give her her bath on one very rare occasion, she asked, "Are you well enough, Mummy?"

~ ~ ~ ~ ~ ~ ~

Today I feel exceptionally good. I take the children to the park. It's only the second time this year, and it's September. The last time, months ago, my husband took us.

The children have been given VERY STRICT instructions not to make it hard for Mummy, when it's time to come home. They understand that if Mummy has to wrestle them into the car, we will not be going again, and if Mummy has to telephone Daddy for help, there will be no chicken for dinner. They agree to anything, for the chance to be out.

~~~~~~~

We go in the car even though the park is just behind our house. I spend the whole time sitting on the bench, flopped over onto the wooden picnic table.

My little girl tries to get into the swing but it's above her head. Her brother, seven years of age, tries to lift her in and fails. I watch and will a nearby parent to lift her in. She doesn't.

They run off and play on the spinning roundabout, then they try again at the swing. This time they succeed. My son gets kicked in the face every time the swing comes back, but he does his best to push his sister. Because I'm not there to supervise, my little girl gets smacked in the face on the rebound when coming off the swing. I watch as she wails in pain.

She pulls herself together and runs off to play again. She climbs into a tree. She walks on a log and speaks to a group of strangers. After a while, I send her brother to check that she is ok. By this time she is shouting for him. The strangers have left and perhaps she realises she's alone.

I watch as they run together to the zip wire in the distance, her little head temporarily disappearing behind a man-made hill. Later they come back and tell me my son has been pushing my daughter on the zip wire. I don't know how she got onto it. Perhaps that is just as well.

My little girl takes food from strangers. From where I sit, I can see it's another parent. My son sports an alarming bruise on his left cheek, which over the course of the evening, will grow to one and a half inches in size. I tell him he's been very brave, and how proud I am of him for looking after his sister. When it's time to go home, their behaviour is exemplary.

~~~~~~~

Several things happen too close together, and now I'm suffering a downturn. I am not supposed to leave the house, even if it's just for a walk round my little cul de sac, any more than once a week. Usually, far, far less. Now I must rest and hope I don't crash. I am unlikely to make it to the park again this year.

My Family

Such a devastating illness affects EVERYONE around you. From anxiety to grief, anger to understanding, attitudes and priorities to psychological and financial issues, the adjustments are massive. Friends are lost, new friends are made. The world shrinks. Then it grows again in a different direction.

Your extended family have to pull together. Your colleagues have to fill the gap you leave, and your friends have to accommodate your new "normal". Some people have to be removed from your life altogether!

With ME/CFS, there is no choice in the matter. When a person is so draining of energy that just having them as an active contact on your phone, never knowing when a message might come in, turns your body into jelly and your knees into mush, and keeps you bedridden all day, there is no option but to remove that person from your life.

If you are lucky, people act with love for your children. But disbelief and dismissal is common. Our illness does not show outwardly, and our disability is invisible.

Perhaps the wider story will one day be the subject of another book. For now, here are some photographs of those dear to me, the people most affected by my illness.

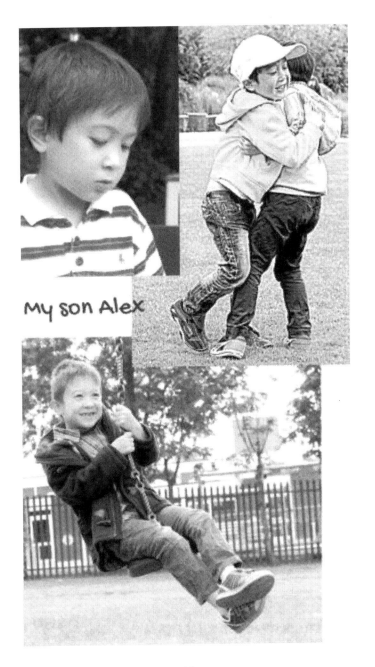

My son Alex

Alex
and
me

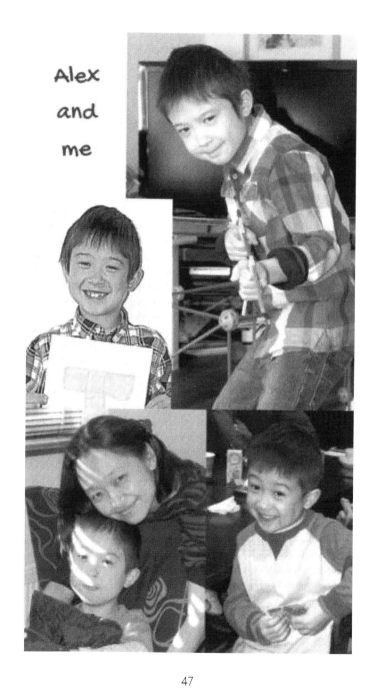

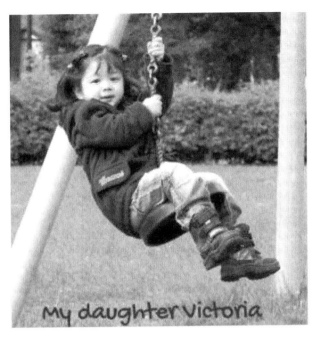

My daughter Victoria

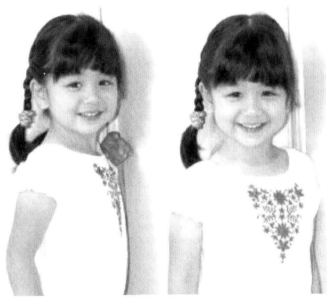

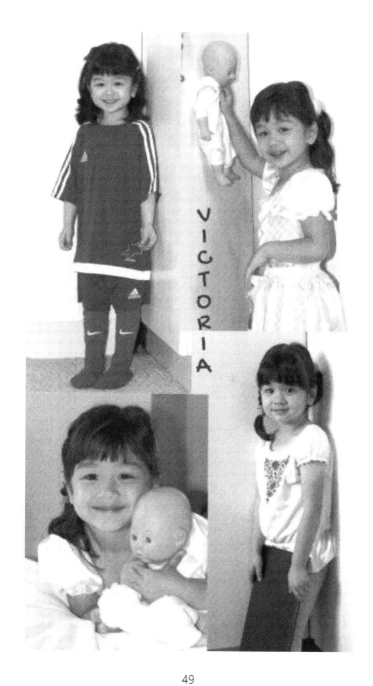

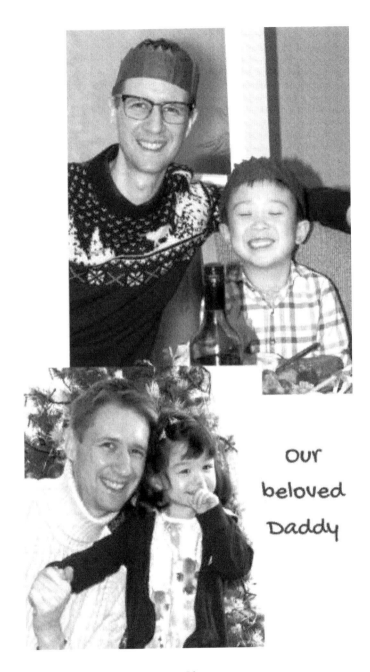

Our beloved Daddy

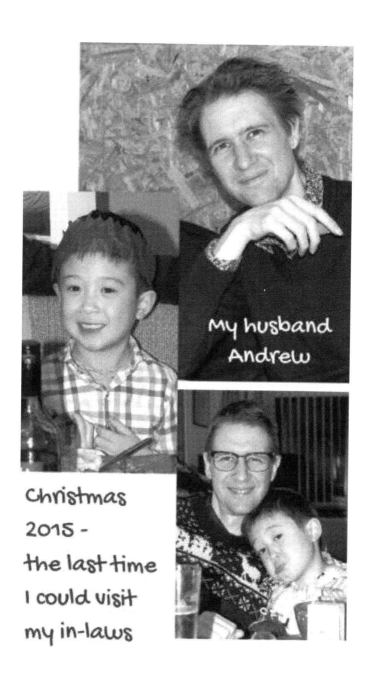

My husband
Andrew

Christmas
2015 –
the last time
I could visit
my in-laws

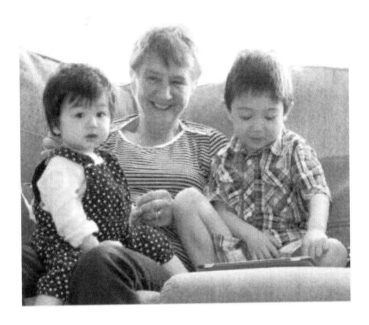

Granny

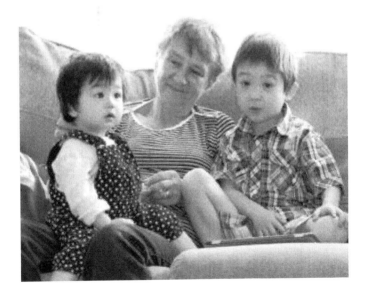

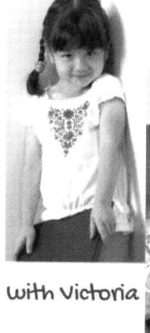

Neighbour
Marion

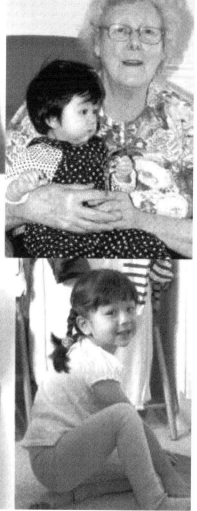

With Victoria

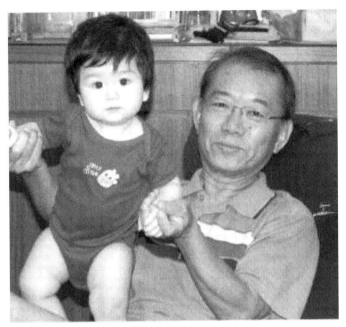

My dear Father
With baby Victoria

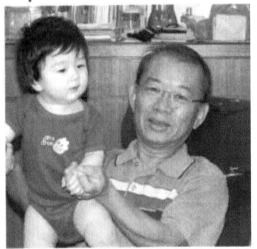

Last seen
Victoria
in 2015,
last seen
Alex in
Aug 2013.
It's now
October
2017.

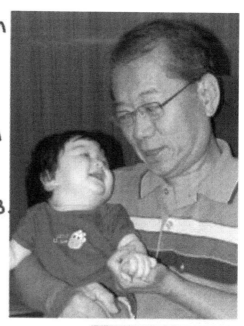

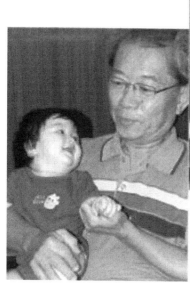

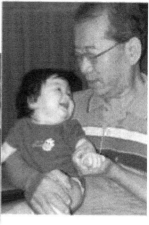

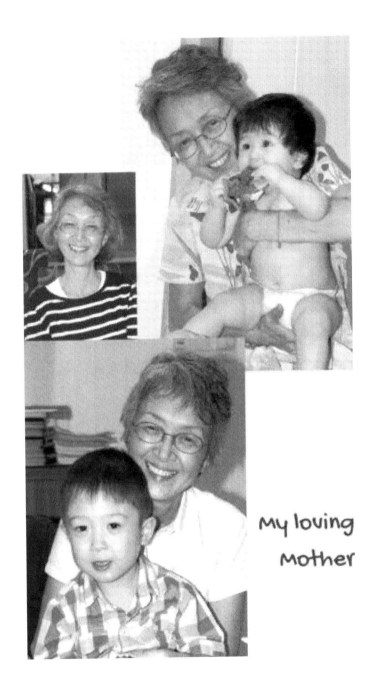

My loving
Mother

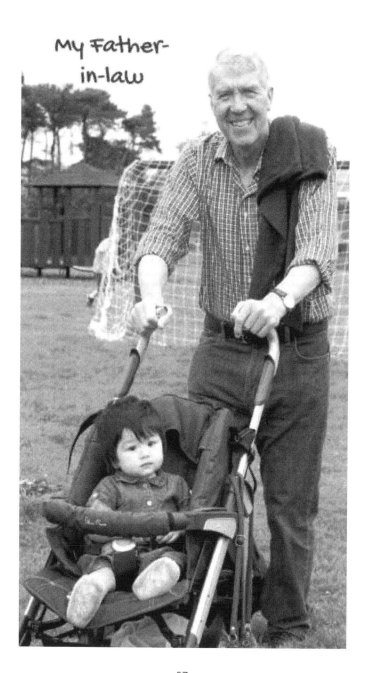

My Father-
in-law

Invisible

When neighbours no longer saw me do my walks around our street, they assumed I had gone back to work. In actual fact I had crashed and was stuck in my bed. At work, despite feeling dreadful, I looked so normal that none of the dozens of doctors I worked with even considered that I might be ill.

Nobody sees us when we are down. When we are better and we do the few things that we can do, be it a little housework or some grocery shopping, we look well, and no one has any idea of the exhaustion that follows, or the hours spent in bed in between. Last week I accompanied my son to the Young Harps workshop at the Royal Northern College of Music. My husband drove, and apart from the last 20 minutes when I watched my son perform with the other children, I spent the morning sleeping on a bench. Even so, upon returning home I had to spend all afternoon in bed, and I didn't brush my teeth at all that day. I also skipped my shower for the third day in a row.

If we have visitors, we rest for days beforehand in preparation, and our visitors see us interacting with them. But once they are gone, we pay the price, taking days or weeks to recover. Again, nobody knows the sacrifice it takes to be able to see our friends once in a blue moon, the debilitation we live with, the choices we make. The world only sees us when we are functional.

I can't remember when I last went to the dentist or the hairdresser.

Across the globe, thousands of young people spend all their days in a quiet, darkened room, unable to tolerate any sensory stimulation. Some are unable to even feed themselves, while others move only by dragging their rag doll bodies across the floor in their homes. With years of suffering and no end in sight many have committed suicide, and experts report excessive deaths from cancer and heart failure.[†]

Yet the medical community is largely ignorant of the magnitude of our suffering, the extent of our disability, the seriousness and multi-system nature of our illness, the multiplicity of our symptoms, and our physical pain. When we are too unwell we can't get to the doctor, and when we do go to them we look completely normal and all standard tests are negative.

The doctor doesn't see me crawl on the floor. The doctor doesn't know I don't shower every day or brush my teeth twice a day like everyone else. He isn't aware of my frequent sore throats, my poor balance, my difficulties with reading, my muscle twitches, or my sound intolerance, and he certainly wasn't here to nurse me when once I was too weak to eat.

The confusing, trivialising and inappropriate name for the condition "Chronic Fatigue Syndrome" further serves to reinforce the impression that there is nothing really wrong. Effectively, we are invisible.

Many patients are misdiagnosed with a psychological illness such as depression or told that it's all in their heads. This is not only unhelpful but actually harmful. It robs patients of the option of the right management, and a psychological approach of "positive thinking", encouraging patients to ignore their symptoms and carry on with activity, or even to exercise, is the most harmful intervention possible. The damage can be great and many patients never recover. In the misguided pursuit of psychological or psychiatric cures, some patients have even been incarcerated in mental institutions!

The situation is even more shocking with children.

Dr Nigel Speight, Consultant Pediatrician with great experience with ME/CFS, states that across the country, child protection proceedings have been instigated against parents trying to protect their sick children from forced harmful treatments. Many children have been removed from their caring homes and placed into hospitals and institutions where they have been systematically abused by well-meaning professionals intent on forcing them to exercise. Needless to say, these children only get sicker, and are severely traumatised!

Rest and pacing of activities is EXTREMELY important, in the management of this illness. It is the mainstay of treatment for sadly, even when a patient is taken seriously and given the right diagnosis, there is no effective cure the doctors can offer. For decades this invisible illness has had little attention from the scientific and research community, and our understanding of its causation, let alone potential treatments, is glaringly scant. However, following prolonged investigative and advocacy efforts by multiple individuals and patient groups, there is now finally some hope that the tide is beginning to turn.

---

† The National Alliance for Myalgic Encephalomyelitis, at: http://www.name-us.org (accessed 19 Oct 2017).

For proper research on ME/CFS, please support
1. The End ME/CFS Project:
   https://www.omf.ngo/the-end-mecfs-project/
2. Invest in ME Research:
   http://www.investinme.org/index.shtml

A New Project

In my exile, I began to explore my creativity. The children and I played with loom bands and Hama beads. I took photos and videos of them. Before I was properly diagnosed, the Occupational Health doctor had said I had "work related stress", and recommended a healthy dose of child's play! And it really did feel good "wasting time" doing things just because they were fun, like making a whole fleet of multi-coloured seahorses!

At one point, I started playing the piano. It took many, many months of repeated crashes and eventually learning to remain housebound in order to keep things more stable, before I could do that. I could only play for very short periods. Half an hour would be too long. All my energy would be spent, I would become very weak, and have to rest in bed. Since my last crash, I have not been able to play again, though I continue to wait patiently for the day I get strong enough once more.

Eventually my attention turned to the coloured music sheets that I had made for my son over the years. I decided to do them properly on the computer, as I needed more music for the children. Soon I found myself writing some very easy lessons to go with the music, with other parents in mind.

Publication was a pie in the sky, but I carried on. I couldn't help myself, for I am a teacher at heart. Teaching was the one area at work in which I still excelled, even as I lived through hell not knowing I was ill.

Now the ideas kept coming. I wrote progressive lessons and arranged the music around them, filling eight books. And I'm still not done.

The teacher in me is calling out. This is such a fun

and easy way for beginners to play music, I want all children, and any adult who has always wished they could play, to try it!

There is no need to worry about music lessons. Unlike other music books, my books are meant to be used at home by parents rather than by music teachers, though several music teachers have expressed an interest! They are a great way to start for anyone uncertain about the commitment to formal lessons. Even for those who never intend to take lessons, they form a large bank of easy fun.

I am now pleased to be able to announce that the first book in the series has been published! It is called "Fun Piano for Children" and can be found on Amazon. The rest of the series will follow.

One day I will come back to work. Until then, wish me luck with my new venture!

The End

Epilogue

Dear reader, thank you so much for reading my book. I hope it has been useful to you. I have just one more thing to say about this. That is, I am classed as a moderate case. I leave you to imagine what a severe case is like. If you are a patient, or a relative or friend of one, you may already know!

The 2011 International Consensus Criteria (see link below) provides the following grades of severity:

Mild – approximately 50% reduction in activity

Moderate – mostly housebound

Severe – mostly bedridden

Very severe – totally bedridden and need help
with basic functions.

If you would like to learn more about this illness, here are some illuminating documentaries:

- **Unrest** by Jennifer Brea (more a movie than a documentary but has been very well received)
- **What about ME?** by Susan Douglas
- **Forgotten Plague** by Ryan Prior
- **Voices from the Shadows** by Natalie Boulton and Josh Biggs
- **Perversely Dark** by Pal Winsents
- **Invisible** by The Vermont CFIDS Association
- **I Remember Me** by Kim A. Snyder

To further the cause for all ME/CFS sufferers, please consider buying several extra copies of this book, to be given to doctors, libraries, medical schools, hospitals, or politicians. Together we can raise awareness of the realities of this illness, educate, and encourage proper research. If you know any organisations which are willing to sponsor wider dissemination, please ask them to get in touch at RColourMusic@hotmail.com. Please also write a review of the book on Amazon. This will increase its visibility to potential buyers.

Afterword

ME or CFS?

The names Myalgic Encephalomyelitis and Chronic Fatigue Syndrome are used interchangeably in this book, as they are in many places, but there is great controversy over what the correct name should be, with accusations of deliberate fudging by rogue organisations and individuals. To add to the confusion, many other names have been or are still used, and there are at present several different official diagnostic criteria.

I do not claim to know the entire history and evolution of the name(s) of this illness, nor have I scrutinised all the research, but discussion with experts in the field tell me the following:

What is clear is that ME/CFS is not a psychological or

mental illness, a neurosis, or behavioural problem. It is an organic disease, with identifiable and measurable pathology. Accordingly, the previously recommended psychological treatments of Cognitive Behavioural Therapy (CBT) and Graded Exercise Therapy (GET) are ineffective,[1] and indeed GET is particularly dangerous.[2]

The use of the name Chronic Fatigue Syndrome has confused clinicians and trivialised the illness. The fact that chronic fatigue is very common indeed, in many physical, psychiatric and other conditions, and is so easily confused with Chronic Fatigue Syndrome, has greatly contributed to a lack of understanding. As a clinical descriptor CFS is hopelessly inadequate. This illness is so much more than just fatigue. It is a serious multi-system neuro-immune condition.

Some diagnostic criteria are not specific enough, and if patients with other causes of fatigue are included, research becomes meaningless. Robust research is needed, and effective treatments found, for a patient population which has been left suffering, ignored and neglected for far too long.

One contemporary and very informative diagnostic criteria is the 2011 International Consensus Criteria, which can be found here:

http://www.meassociation.org.uk/2011/07/myalgic-encephalomyelitis-international-consensus-criteria-journal-of-internal-medicine-20-july-2011/

The following websites provide much useful information:

http://www.name-us.org

http://www.meassociation.org.uk/me-association/

And this is an eye-opening piece of investigative journalism:

https://undark.org/article/chronic-fatigue-graded-exercise-pace/

Harmful Psychological "Treatments"

Unbelievably, even in the present day, psychological "treatments" are being developed and promoted for ME/CFS, which tell patients to "think" their symptoms away, alarmingly encouraging them to push beyond their limits, and blaming the patients themselves for not trying hard enough, when they worsen or do not improve! I urge all my readers to be extremely wary of any treatment which uses a "mind over matter" approach and tells you not to listen to your body. Even where clinical trial data is cited, I urge you to examine the evidence for yourself and read widely about a proposed treatment before making your decision. Ask yourself the following questions about any clinical trial:

1. Did they recruit the right patients? Or is their entry criteria so loose that they could have recruited patients who actually have depression or anxiety rather than ME/CFS? Remember many

conditions can cause the "six months of fatigue" used in weak diagnostic criteria.

2. Where did the study patients come from? Were they a captive audience that could have been easily manipulated, for example patients attending the clinic of the chief investigator who hopes to gain financially from a particular treatment? Is there a selection bias? For example, if only a minority of the patients approached agreed to participate in a study, what separates those who agreed and those who did not? The difference could be that some are real ME/CFS patients who know from experience that a proposed treatment would be harmful, while others are actually "fatigue" patients who may have a large psychological component or other factors.

3. What is the end point being studied? For example, this could mean return to work,

improvement in function, or psychological effects. Is it an objective, measurable endpoint, or a subjective, self-reported one? The latter is completely meaningless when a psychological approach or brainwashing method is being studied, where participants are programmed to report positive answers.

4. Did the study measure the originally intended endpoint, or was the end point slackened along the way to produce the desired trial result?

5. If a trial reports a positive result, is it truly a positive result for ME/CFS, or is it inapplicable to ME/CFS because of meaningless entry criteria (see point 1) and selection bias (see point 2)? Is the chosen end point a meaningful one (see point 3)? And is the result based on the originally chosen end point (see point 4), or merely a modified version that was designed to produce a positive result?

6. And finally, is there any potential conflict of interest, such as a commercial treatment which costs large sums of money? Sadly, not all conflicts of interest are transparently declared with reported studies as they ought to be, or properly explained to participants before a study as they should be.

One example of a very badly conducted clinical trial which to me, appears to have been designed to produce the desired result, is critiqued here by the ME Association:

http://www.meassociation.org.uk/2017/10/mea-review-the-smile-trial-a-lesson-in-how-not-to-conduct-clinical-trials-in-people-with-mecfs-12-october-2017/

Useful Psychological Approach[3]

This is not to say that dealing with psychological issues has no place in the management of ME/CFS. With such profound losses and little medical help available, patients have much to contend with. In addition, patients face disbelief and dismissal, and are burdened by guilt over what they can't do, especially those who have children.

Psychological stress and negative feelings such as anger, frustration and guilt saps energy. With no energy left over for healing, a patient's body cannot begin to recover. Therefore work around acceptance of the situation and dealing with expectations would be beneficial.

Patients also need to learn how to stay within one's limits – a technique called "pacing". Work to deal with any other issues patients may have in their lives, or changes in roles and relationships, so that they can be freed from any chains that bind them and hold them back, would also be useful.

References:

1. Vincent Racaniello, (2016) "No 'Recovery' in PACE Trial, New Analysis Finds", in *Virology Blog*, 21 Sep 2016.
    Available at: http://www.virology.ws/2016/09/21/no-recovery-in-pace-trial-new-analysis-finds/ (Accessed: 28 Sep 2017).

2. David Tuller, (2016) "Worse Than the Disease", in *Undark: Truth, Beauty, Science.* 27 Oct 2016.
    Available at: https://undark.org/article/chronic-fatigue-graded-exercise-pace/ (Accessed: 28 Sep 2017).

3. Personal opinion.

Acknowledgements

I am grateful to my editor, Milton Trachtenburg, a master psychotherapist, writer, and a wise old friend.

Thank you to Helen Pryke for proof-reading, and to the countless individuals who have furnished me with resources and/or helped with the design of my book cover. Special thanks to those who have directly influenced the contents of this book, though many of you won't know it.

Finally, all my love to my wonderful family, who make it all worthwhile, and who make it all possible.

About the Author

Dr Hng is a Gastroenterology trainee in the United Kingdom. Her credentials includes her basic medical degree MBChB, Membership of the Royal College of Physicians (MRCP), Postgraduate Certificate in Work Based Medical Education (PGCert in WBME), and Fellowship of the Higher Education Authority (FHEA).

Dr Hng excels as a teacher. She was previously a Teaching Fellow, and later an Honorary Lecturer, at the Manchester Medical School, one of the largest in the country. She is the named author of its Year 3 Liver, Biliary and Pancreatic Diseases online module.

Musically, Dr Hng is trained to ABRSM Grade 7 on the piano. If you would like to explore her music books, please visit:

https://www.facebook.com/RColourMusic/

Music Books Preview:

Capture the interest of young children with these brightly coloured notes!

- Play tunes right away.

- No knowledge needed – just follow the

  colours.

- Fun exercises.

- Solfege – develops the ability to play by ear.

- One simple lesson in each book.

- Correct musical notation

  – for easy transition to formal lessons.

- Can be used with some other instruments

  – guitar, plucked strings, xylophone.

- Written for parents.

Alex's Story

Alex was a shy little boy who was always singing. When he was very little, his Mummy put coloured dots on her piano, and wrote out some of his favourite songs in coloured notes. Alex was able to play these songs by following the colours. Soon he was playing dozens of songs, and asking for more! By the time Alex was 5 years old, he was good enough that his school was persuaded to provide formal piano lessons. Before long he was performing at school events, and he continues to enjoy learning and playing the piano today.

Now you, too, can introduce your child to the delights of playing music. This imaginative book series captures the interest of very young children by being so easy to follow, even before a child can read or write. The bright colours and instant audible result of their efforts is sure to keep them coming back for more!